Rice Toner 101: Quick Facts for Glowing Skin

Your Comprehensive Handbook for Healthy Skin and Rice Toners

A J BLAZE

DISCLAIMER

The book Rice Toner 101: Quick Facts for Glowing Skin provides information and insight on the benefits of incorporating rice toner into your skincare routine. The content contained herein is for general information purposes only and should not be considered professional advice. Skincare recommendations and practices may vary depending on your individual needs, skin type, and health. Readers are encouraged to seek individual advice from a qualified medical or skin care professional. People with allergies or skin sensitivities should use caution when trying new skincare methods or products. The DIY skin care recipes provided in this book are shared as suggestions and readers should be aware of their own skin's reactions. It is important to follow good hygiene practices when creating and using homemade skin care products. The results mentioned herein are general and may not apply to everyone. Any specific product recommendations mentioned herein are for illustrative purposes only and do not constitute recommendations. Readers should conduct their research and consider their skin conditions before selecting skin care products. For additional information, this document may contain references to external websites. The inclusion of these links does not constitute an endorsement, and the authors are not responsible for the content, accuracy, or security of external websites. Readers are responsible for their own skincare choices and practices. When implementing a new skincare routine, it's important to be aware of your skin conditions, allergies, and preferences. We encourage our readers to stay informed as their skin care practices evolve. By reading this book, readers acknowledge that they are responsible for their own skincare choices and should consult a qualified professional if necessary.

Contents

Introduction 13

the concept of rice toner. 13

Popularity In Skincare Routines. 14

The Quick Facts to Be Covered. 15

The Origins: 15

Science Behind the Glow: 15

Diverse Benefits: 15

Types of Rice Toners 16

DIY Delights: 16

Application Mastery: 16

Choosing the Perfect Fit 16

Recap and Reinforce: 17

Chapter 1 19

The Basics of Rice Toner 19

1.1 The Origin and History of Rice Toner. ...19

1.2 The Science Behind Its Effectiveness. ...21

Moisture Retention: 22

Skin Brightening Enzymes: 22

Soothing and Calming Properties:.......... 22

Chapter 2 25

Benefits for Your Skin 25

2.1 The Various Benefits of Using Rice Toner.

.... 25

Radiant Complexion: 25

Hydration Boost:...................................... 26

Antioxidant Defense: 26

Soothing and Calming: 26

Even Skin Tone: 26

Versatility for All Skin Types: 27

Prepares Skin for Further Products: 27

Natural and Gentle: 27

2.2 The Brightening, Moisturizing, And Antioxidant Properties. 28

Brightening Properties: 28

Moisturizing Efficacy: 29

Antioxidant Defense: 29

Chapter 3 31

Types of Rice Toners 31

3.1 The Different Types of Rice Toners Available in The Market. 31

Traditional Rice Water Toners: 31

Rice Bran Extract Toners:........................ 32

Fermented Rice Toners: 32

Rice Extract Infused Toners: 33

Rice Oil-Infused Toners:......................... 33

Multi-Ingredient Rice Toners:................. 33

Sheet Mask Rice Toners:......................... 34

3.2 Insights into Their Specific Uses and Formulations. 35

1. Traditional Rice Water Toners:........... 35

2. Rice Bran Extract Toners:................... 35

3. Fermented Rice Toners: 36

4. Rice Extract Infused Toners: 36

5. Rice Oil-Infused Toners:..................... 37

6. Multi-Ingredient Rice Toners:........... 37

7. Sheet Mask Rice Toners:.....................38

Chapter 4 39

DIY Rice Toner Recipes.................................. 39

4.1 Simple and Effective Recipes for Making
Rice Toner at Home................................... 39

Recipe 1: Basic Rice Water Toner 39

Recipe 2: Rice and Green Tea Toner 41

4.2 Variations for Different Skin Types...... 42

Recipe 1: Basic Rice Water Toner 42

For Dry Skin:... 42

For Oily or Acne-Prone Skin:.................. 43

For Sensitive Skin: 43

Recipe 2: Rice and Green Tea Toner 43

For Dry or Mature Skin: 43

For Oily or Acne-Prone Skin:.................. 44

For Sensitive Skin: 44

Chapter 5 45

Application Tips and Techniques................... 45

5.1 Practical Tips for Incorporating Rice
Toner into A Skincare Routine. 45

Cleanse First: 45

Use a Cotton Pad or Hands:.................... 46

Focus on Problem Areas: 46

Morning and Night Application: 46

Follow with Serum or Moisturizer: 47

DIY Sheet Mask: 47

Refrigerate for a Refreshing Experience 47

Customize According to Seasons:............ 48

Observe Your Skin's Response: 48

Consistency is Key: 48

5.2 Guidance on When and How to Apply It for Optimal Results.................................... 49

When to Apply Rice Toner:...................... 49

Morning Routine: 49

Evening Routine: 50

After Cleansing:....................................... 50

Before Serum or Moisturizer: 50

Throughout the Day (Optional):.............. 50

How to Apply Rice Toner:........................51

Pour onto a Cotton Pad:............................51

Swipe Gently Across Face: 51

Pat onto Skin (Alternative): 51

DIY Sheet Mask (Optional): 51

Avoid Eye Area:.. 52

Follow with Other Skincare Products:.... 52

Store Properly: 52

Be Consistent: 52

Chapter 6 55

Choosing the Right Rice Toner for Your Skin
Type 55

6.1 Selecting the Most Suitable Rice Toner
Based on Their Skin Type............................ 55

1. For Dry Skin: 55

2. For Oily or Acne-Prone Skin:............... 56

3. For Combination Skin:......................... 56

4. For Sensitive Skin: 57

5. For Aging or Mature Skin: 57

6. For Dull or Uneven Skin Tone:............57

General Tips for All Skin Types: 58

6.2 common concerns and considerations. 59

1. Allergies and Sensitivities: 60

2. Acne and Breakouts: 60

3. Over-Exfoliation: 60

4. Hydration Levels: 61

5. Choosing the Right Type: 61

6. Patch Testing: 62

7. Storage and Shelf Life: 62

8. Consistency in Usage 62

9. Potential for Irritation: 63

10. Adapting to Seasonal Changes: 63

Chapter 7 65

Quick Facts Recap 65

7.1 The Key Quick Facts Presented in This Book. 65

Conclusion 69

The Importance of Incorporating Rice Toner into A Skincare Routine 69

Radiant Complexion: 69

Hydration Boost:.................................. 70

Antioxidant Defense: 70

Soothing and Calming: 70

Even Skin Tone: 71

Versatility for All Skin Types: 71

Prepares Skin for Further Products: 71

Natural and Gentle: 72

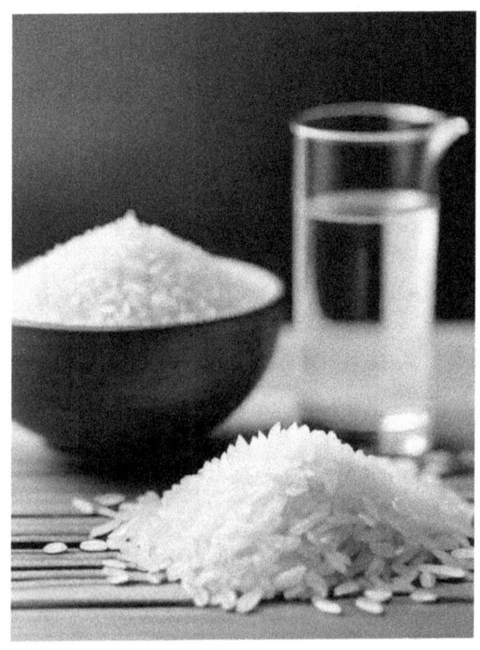

Introduction
the concept of rice toner.

Rice toner is a skincare product that harnesses the natural properties of rice extract or rice water to benefit the skin. This concept draws inspiration from traditional beauty practices, particularly in Asian cultures, where rice has been used for centuries for its potential skincare advantages.

Rice toner is known for its brightening effects, moisturizing properties, and antioxidant content, making it a popular choice for those seeking a natural and gentle addition to their skincare routine.

The toner is believed to contribute to a more radiant complexion, even skin tone, and overall skin health. With both commercial products and DIY recipes available, rice toner has gained recognition for its versatility and potential benefits for various skin types.

Popularity In Skincare Routines.

Rice toner has surged in popularity within skincare routines, becoming a favored choice among beauty enthusiasts. Its rise to prominence is attributed to its natural and gentle approach to skincare, offering users a botanical alternative to traditional toners. As an integral part of skincare regimens, rice toner is celebrated for its ability to impart a radiant glow, even out skin tone, and contribute to a healthier complexion. Its widespread adoption showcases a growing acknowledgment of the beneficial properties that rice toner brings to modern skincare practices.

The Quick Facts to Be Covered.

In "Rice Toner 101: Quick Facts for Glowing Skin," we'll explore a wealth of information aimed at enhancing your understanding and appreciation of rice toner in skincare. Here's a sneak peek at the quick facts we'll be covering:

The Origins: Delve into the historical roots of rice toner, understanding how ancient beauty practices inspired its modern use.

Science Behind the Glow: Uncover the scientific principles that make rice toner a powerhouse in skincare, from brightening effects to antioxidant-rich formulations.

Diverse Benefits: Explore the multifaceted benefits of rice toner, including its capacity to moisturize, soothe, and contribute to a more even skin tone.

Types of Rice Toners: Navigate the diverse landscape of rice toner products, discovering variations in formulations and identifying the most suitable options for your skincare needs.

DIY Delights: Unlock the secrets of creating your own rice toner at home with simple and effective DIY recipes, tailored to different skin types.

Application Mastery: Learn practical tips and techniques for seamlessly integrating rice toner into your daily skincare routine, maximizing its benefits for radiant and healthy skin.

Choosing the Perfect Fit: Gain insights into selecting the right rice toner based on your unique skin type, addressing common concerns and optimizing results.

Recap and Reinforce: Summarize the key quick facts, reinforcing the compelling reasons to make rice toner a staple in your skincare regimen.

Join us on this journey as we demystify the world of rice toner, empowering you with knowledge to achieve that coveted glowing and healthy skin.

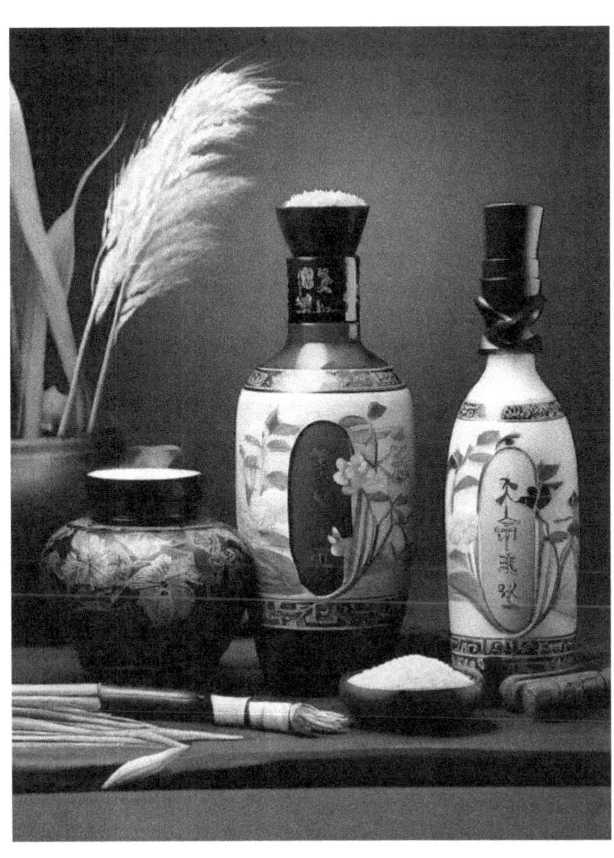

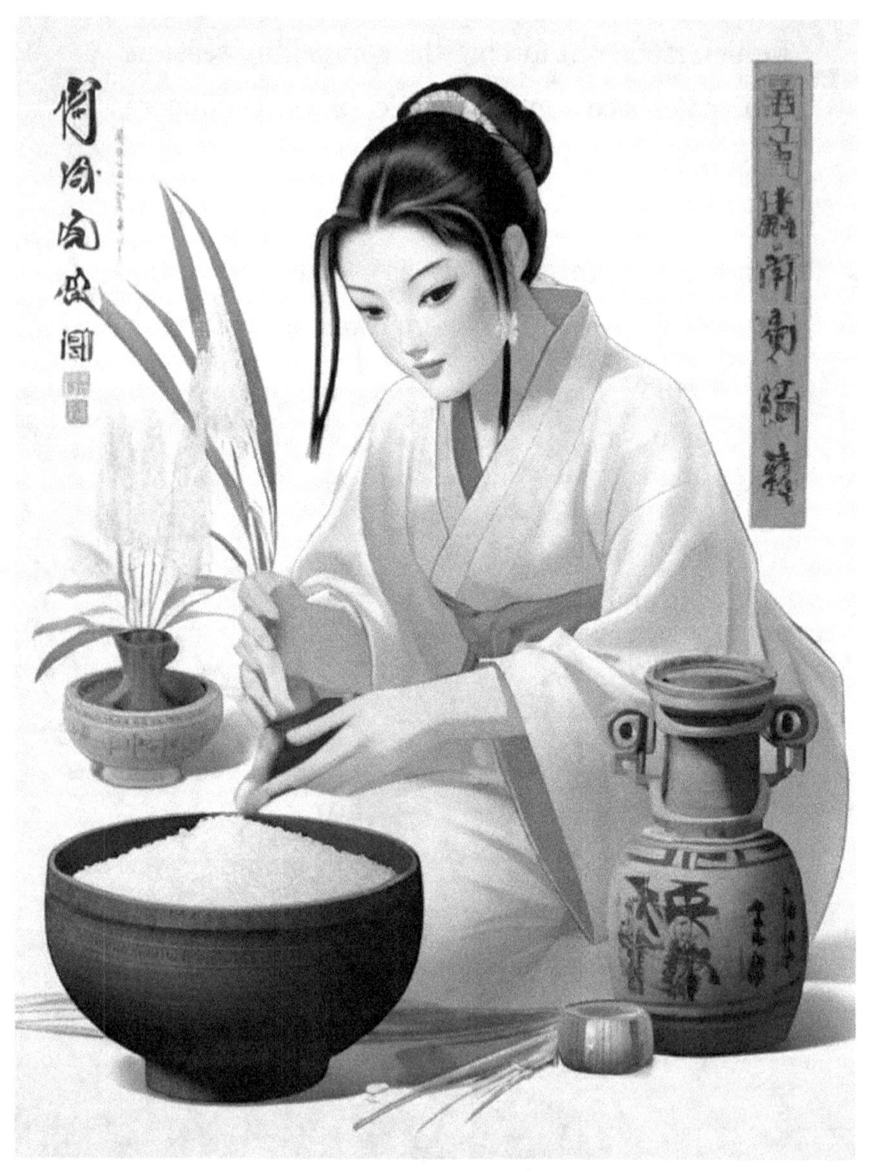

Chapter 1
The Basics of Rice Toner

1.1 The Origin and History of Rice Toner.

The exploration of the origin and history of rice toner unveils a fascinating narrative rooted in ancient beauty practices and cultural traditions. Dating back centuries, particularly in Asian cultures, rice has been revered not only as a dietary staple but also for its transformative properties in skincare rituals.

The historical application of rice water, a byproduct of rinsing rice during cooking, emerged as a natural elixir for promoting skin health. Esteemed for its gentle yet effective qualities, rice water was traditionally used by individuals seeking to enhance the clarity and luminosity of their skin.

Over time, this practice evolved, and the concept of rice toner emerged as a refined skincare product. As beauty traditions transcended borders, rice toner gained international recognition, securing its place as a coveted component within modern skincare routines.

The contemporary formulation of rice toner blends time-honored wisdom with advanced skincare science, offering users a sophisticated solution for achieving radiant and balanced skin. This journey into the origin and history of rice toner underscores its enduring appeal, illustrating how an age-old practice has seamlessly integrated into the dynamic landscape of today's skincare industry.

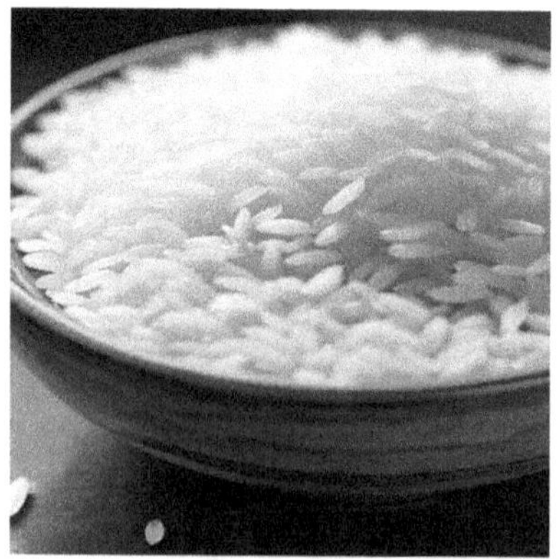

1.2 The Science Behind Its Effectiveness.

Understanding the science behind the effectiveness of rice toner requires a closer examination of the intricate components inherent in this skincare elixir. Rice, a staple with a rich history in beauty traditions, boasts a profile that aligns seamlessly with the principles of skincare science.

Nutrient-Rich Composition: Rice is inherently rich in vitamins, minerals, and amino acids. These nutritional elements contribute to the nourishment and revitalization of the skin, promoting a healthy complexion.

Antioxidant Properties: The presence of antioxidants in rice toner helps combat free radicals, the unstable molecules responsible for oxidative stress and premature aging. This defensive mechanism assists in preserving the skin's youthful appearance.

Moisture Retention: Rice toner's moisturizing efficacy is attributed to its ability to lock in hydration. The natural components in rice form a protective barrier on the skin, preventing moisture loss and fostering a supple and hydrated complexion.

Skin Brightening Enzymes: Some formulations of rice toner include enzymes that contribute to gentle exfoliation. This process helps remove dead skin cells, unveiling a brighter and more even skin tone over time.

Soothing and Calming Properties: Rice toner is known for its soothing effects on the skin. Whether addressing irritation or redness, the calming properties of rice toner make it a preferred choice for those with sensitive skin.

By merging traditional wisdom with scientific understanding, rice toner emerges as a skincare ally, its effectiveness grounded in a nuanced interplay of botanical elements.

This amalgamation showcases the product's ability to align with the principles of modern skincare science, offering users a holistic solution for achieving radiant and healthy skin.

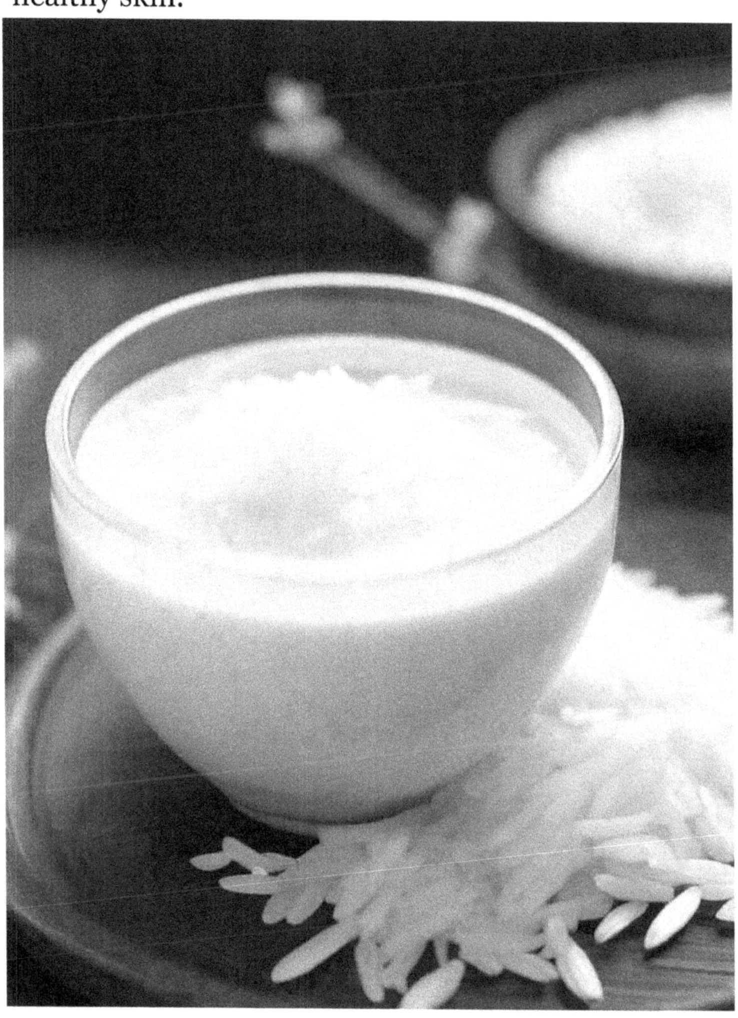

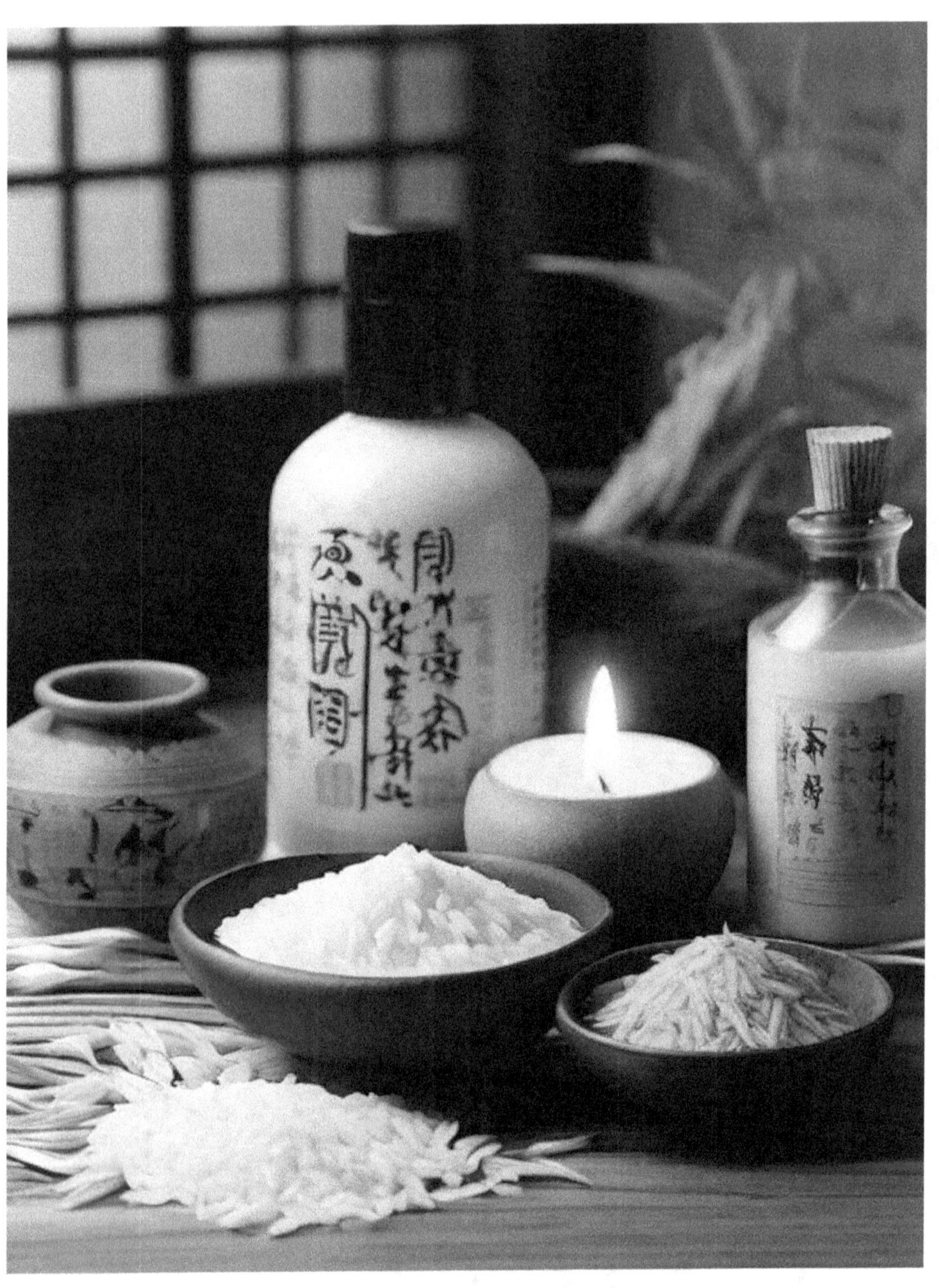

Chapter 2
Benefits for Your Skin

2.1 The Various Benefits of Using Rice Toner.

Embracing the use of rice toner in your skincare routine offers a myriad of benefits, elevating it to a coveted position among beauty enthusiasts. Here's a spotlight on the various advantages that make rice toner a transformative addition to your regimen:

Radiant Complexion: Rice toner is renowned for its brightening properties, contributing to a luminous and radiant complexion. Regular use helps diminish dullness, leaving your skin with a healthy glow.

Hydration Boost: The natural moisturizing elements in rice toner aid in restoring and maintaining optimal skin hydration. This makes it an excellent choice for individuals seeking a lightweight yet effective solution for dry or dehydrated skin.

Antioxidant Defense: Packed with antioxidants, rice toner acts as a formidable defense against free radicals. This helps protect the skin from environmental stressors, reducing the risk of premature aging and maintaining a youthful appearance.

Soothing and Calming: Ideal for sensitive skin, rice toner's soothing properties alleviate irritation and redness. It provides a gentle and calming effect, making it suitable for individuals with various skin sensitivities.

Even Skin Tone: The potential exfoliating enzymes in rice toner contribute to a smoother and more even skin tone.

This can be particularly beneficial for addressing hyperpigmentation and uneven texture.

Versatility for All Skin Types: Whether you have oily, dry, combination, or sensitive skin, rice toner is known for its versatility. It adapts well to different skin types, offering a universal solution for a diverse range of skincare needs.

Prepares Skin for Further Products: Using rice toner as part of your skincare routine preps the skin by removing impurities and creating a receptive canvas for subsequent products. This enhances the efficacy of serums, moisturizers, and other treatments.

Natural and Gentle: One of the standout features of rice toner is its natural and gentle nature. Free from harsh chemicals, it provides an effective yet mild option for those seeking a botanical approach to skincare.

Incorporating rice toner into your daily routine aligns with a holistic approach to skincare, offering a host of benefits that contribute to a healthier, more vibrant, and resilient complexion.

2.2 The Brightening, Moisturizing, And Antioxidant Properties.

Brightening Properties:

One of the standout benefits of using rice toner lies in its remarkable brightening properties. Rich in vitamins and nutrients, rice toner helps to diminish dullness and uneven skin tone. The natural compounds present in rice contribute to a more luminous complexion, unveiling a radiant and revitalized skin surface.

Moisturizing Efficacy:

Rice toner serves as a potent moisturizer, aiding in the restoration and retention of skin hydration. Its innate ability to lock in moisture makes it an excellent choice for individuals seeking a hydrating solution that is both lightweight and effective. Regular use of rice toner helps maintain supple and nourished skin, preventing dryness and promoting a healthy moisture balance.

Antioxidant Defense:

The antioxidant-rich profile of rice toner makes it a formidable ally in the fight against free radicals. These antioxidants act as protective agents, guarding the skin against environmental stressors that can lead to premature aging. By neutralizing free radicals, rice toner supports the skin's resilience, helping to maintain a youthful and vibrant appearance over time.

Incorporating rice toner into your skincare routine harnesses the combined power of brightening, moisturizing, and antioxidant properties. This trifecta of benefits not only enhances the overall health of your skin but also contributes to a visibly radiant and rejuvenated complexion.

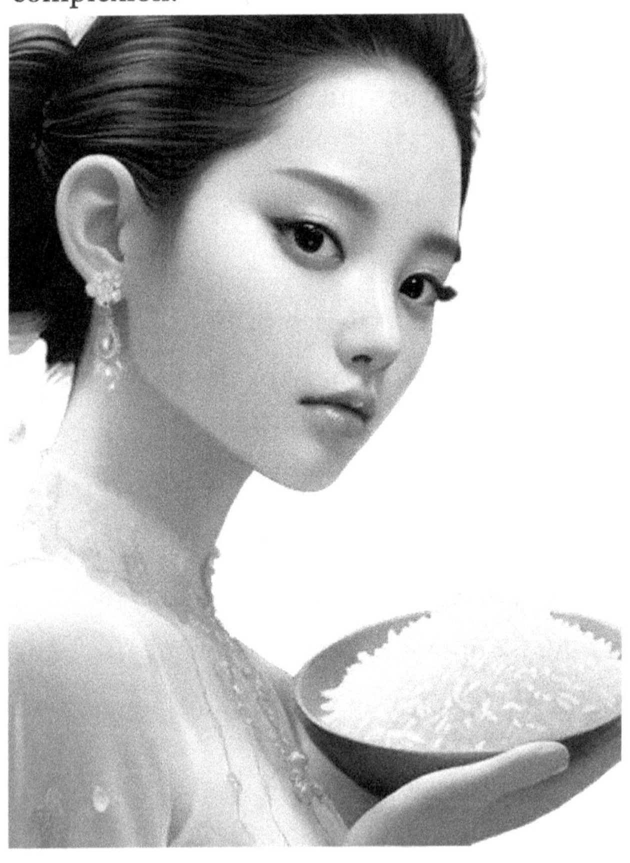

Chapter 3
Types of Rice Toners

3.1 The Different Types of Rice Toners Available in The Market.

The market for rice toners has seen significant diversity, offering consumers various formulations tailored to different skincare needs. Here's an overview of the different types of rice toners available:

Traditional Rice Water Toners:

Derived from the water used to rinse rice during cooking, these toners maintain the simplicity of ancient beauty practices. They often contain natural rice water and are prized for their purity and gentle effects on the skin.

Rice Bran Extract Toners:

Extracted from the outer layer of the rice grain, rice bran toners are rich in vitamins, antioxidants, and fatty acids. These toners contribute to skin nourishment, offering benefits such as moisturization, brightening, and protection against free radicals.

Fermented Rice Toners:

Fermentation processes are employed to enhance the efficacy of rice toners. Fermented rice toners often contain probiotics and enzymes, promoting a healthy skin microbiome. These toners may offer additional benefits such as improved absorption of nutrients and a boost to the skin's natural renewal processes.

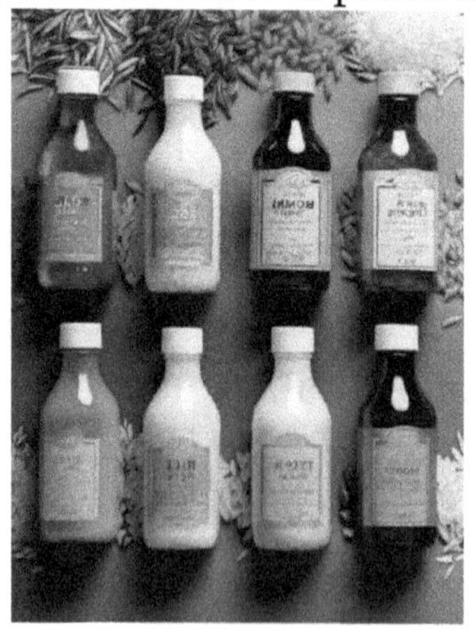

Rice Extract Infused Toners:

Toners infused with concentrated rice extracts deliver a potent dose of nutrients to the skin. These extracts may be combined with other botanical ingredients to create formulations targeting specific skincare concerns, such as anti-aging, brightening, or soothing effects.

Rice Oil-Infused Toners:

Rice oil, extracted from rice bran, is known for its emollient and nourishing properties. Rice oil-infused toners provide deep hydration and can be particularly beneficial for those with dry or mature skin. These toners often leave the skin feeling soft and supple.

Multi-Ingredient Rice Toners:

Combining the benefits of rice with other skincare ingredients, these toners offer a comprehensive approach to skincare.

Formulations may include hyaluronic acid, aloe vera, or other plant extracts to address various skin concerns while leveraging the brightening and moisturizing qualities of rice.

Sheet Mask Rice Toners:

Rice toners are also incorporated into sheet masks, allowing for a convenient and targeted application. These masks typically provide an intense burst of hydration and other benefits, making them a popular choice for a pampering skincare ritual.

Understanding the different types of rice toners enables you to choose products that align with your specific skin needs and preferences. Whether seeking simplicity, fermentation benefits, or a combination of ingredients, the market offers a diverse array of rice toners to cater to individual skincare goals.

3.2 Insights into Their Specific Uses and Formulations.

1. Traditional Rice Water Toners:

Specific Uses: Known for their purity, these toners are gentle and suitable for all skin types. They primarily focus on providing a refreshing and basic level of hydration.

Formulations: Typically contain natural rice water without elaborate additives. Some formulations may include additional soothing ingredients like chamomile or aloe vera.

2. Rice Bran Extract Toners:

Specific Uses: Ideal for those seeking nourishment and anti-aging benefits. Rice bran toners offer deep hydration and work well for addressing uneven skin tone and fine lines.

Formulations: Rich in vitamins, antioxidants, and fatty acids. Formulations may include botanical extracts to enhance the toner's overall skin-rejuvenating properties.

3. Fermented Rice Toners:

Specific Uses: Geared towards promoting a healthy skin microbiome, improving absorption of nutrients, and enhancing skin renewal. Suitable for those seeking overall skin vitality.

Formulations: Utilize fermented rice extracts, probiotics, and enzymes. Additional botanical extracts may be included to amplify the toner's benefits.

4. Rice Extract Infused Toners:

Specific Uses: Versatile and suitable for various skin concerns, including brightening, moisturizing, and soothing. Can be customized based on additional ingredients incorporated into the formulation.

Formulations: Contain concentrated rice extracts along with other botanicals, antioxidants, or humectants to address specific skin needs.

5. Rice Oil-Infused Toners:

Specific Uses: Targeted at providing deep hydration and nourishment, making them ideal for individuals with dry or mature skin.

Formulations: Include rice oil for its emollient properties, and may also incorporate other oils or ingredients for a well-rounded moisturizing effect.

6. Multi-Ingredient Rice Toners:

Specific Uses: Tailored to address a range of skincare concerns such as anti-aging, hydration, and soothing effects.

Formulations: Combine rice extracts with complementary ingredients like hyaluronic acid, aloe vera, or botanical extracts to create a comprehensive skincare solution.

7. Sheet Mask Rice Toners:

Specific Uses: Offer an intense and targeted burst of hydration, making them suitable for a pampering skincare ritual.

Formulations: Typically saturated with a concentrated rice toner solution along with other beneficial ingredients. The sheet mask format enhances absorption and ensures a thorough application.

Understanding the specific uses and formulations of different rice toners enables you to select products that align with your unique skincare goals, whether it be hydration, anti-aging, or overall skin health.

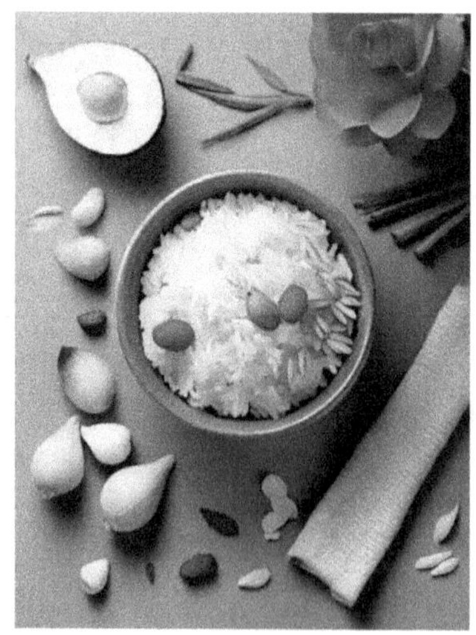

Chapter 4
DIY Rice Toner Recipes

4.1 Simple and Effective Recipes for Making Rice Toner at Home.

Creating a homemade rice toner can be a fun and cost-effective way to incorporate this beneficial skincare ingredient into your routine. Here are two simple and effective recipes for making rice toner at home:

Recipe 1: Basic Rice Water Toner

Ingredients:

1/2 cup uncooked rice (white or brown)

1 cup water

Optional: a few drops of essential oil (e.g., lavender, chamomile) for fragrance

Instructions:

- Rinse the rice thoroughly to remove any impurities.
- Place the rinsed rice in a bowl and add 1 cup of water.
- Let the rice soak in the water for about 15-30 minutes.
- Swirl the rice around in the water, gently pressing it to release its beneficial properties.
- Strain the rice water into a clean container, discarding the rice.
- If desired, add a few drops of your preferred essential oil for fragrance.
- Transfer the rice water toner to a sealed container and store it in the refrigerator for freshness.
- Apply the toner to your face using a cotton pad or by gently patting it onto your skin. Use it after cleansing and before moisturizing.

Recipe 2: Rice and Green Tea Toner

Ingredients:

1/4 cup uncooked rice

1 green tea bag

1 cup water

Optional: aloe vera gel (1-2 tablespoons) for added soothing properties

Instructions:

- Brew a cup of green tea and let it cool to room temperature.
- Rinse the rice thoroughly to remove impurities.
- In a separate bowl, soak the rinsed rice in the green tea for about 30 minutes.
- After soaking, strain the rice and green tea mixture, separating the liquid from the rice.
- If desired, add aloe vera gel to the liquid for additional soothing effects.
- Transfer the toner to a clean container and refrigerate for freshness.

- Apply the toner to your face using a cotton pad or by gently patting it onto your skin. Use it after cleansing and before applying moisturizer.

Remember to perform a patch test before using any homemade skincare products to ensure that your skin reacts well to the ingredients. Store these toners in the refrigerator and use them within a week or two for optimal freshness.

4.2 Variations for Different Skin Types.

Here are variations for the homemade rice toner recipes to suit different skin types:

Recipe 1: Basic Rice Water Toner

For Dry Skin:

- Add 1-2 tablespoons of glycerin to the rice water for extra moisturizing properties.

- Consider using brown rice instead of white rice for added nutrients.

For Oily or Acne-Prone Skin:

- Add 1-2 tablespoons of witch hazel to the rice water for its astringent and acne-fighting properties.
- Include a few drops of tea tree oil for its antibacterial benefits.

For Sensitive Skin:

- Use jasmine rice, known for its calming properties.
- Infuse the rice water with a chamomile tea bag for additional soothing effects.

Recipe 2: Rice and Green Tea Toner

For Dry or Mature Skin:

- Add 1-2 tablespoons of rose water for its hydrating and anti-aging properties.
- Mix in a few drops of argan oil to boost nourishment.

For Oily or Acne-Prone Skin:

- Incorporate 1-2 tablespoons of aloe vera gel for its soothing and anti-inflammatory benefits.
- Consider adding a few drops of lavender oil, known for its antimicrobial properties.

For Sensitive Skin:

- Use green tea with chamomile for a soothing combination.
- Skip the optional aloe vera gel if your skin is highly sensitive.
- Remember to test any new ingredients on a small area of your skin to ensure that they don't cause irritation.
- Adjust the proportions based on your skin's specific needs, and feel free to experiment with different variations until you find the perfect homemade rice toner that suits your skin type.

Chapter 5
Application Tips and Techniques

5.1 Practical Tips for Incorporating Rice Toner into A Skincare Routine.

Incorporating rice toner into your skincare routine is a simple and rewarding process. Here are practical tips to make the most out of this beneficial product:

Cleanse First:

Begin with a gentle cleanser to remove any makeup, dirt, or impurities from your skin before applying the rice toner. This ensures that the toner can be absorbed more effectively.

Use a Cotton Pad or Hands:

Apply the rice toner using a cotton pad to sweep it across your face gently. Alternatively, pour a small amount into clean hands and pat it onto your skin. This allows for even distribution.

Focus on Problem Areas:

Pay extra attention to areas where you may have concerns, such as uneven skin tone or dry patches. Gently pat the toner onto these areas for targeted care.

Morning and Night Application:

Incorporate rice toner into both your morning and evening skincare routines. In the morning, it helps refresh and prepare your skin for makeup application, while at night, it aids in skin repair and rejuvenation.

Follow with Serum or Moisturizer:

After applying the rice toner, follow up with a serum or moisturizer to lock in the benefits and provide additional hydration. This layering technique enhances the overall effectiveness of your skincare routine.

DIY Sheet Mask:

Soak cotton pads or a compressed sheet mask with rice toner and apply it to your face for a DIY sheet mask experience. Leave it on for 10-15 minutes for an extra boost of hydration.

Refrigerate for a Refreshing Experience:

Store your rice toner in the refrigerator for a refreshing sensation during application. The cool temperature can help soothe the skin and reduce puffiness.

Customize According to Seasons:

Adjust the frequency of rice toner use based on the seasons. In drier seasons, you may opt to use it more often for added hydration, while in warmer weather, you might use it to refresh your skin.

Observe Your Skin's Response:

Pay attention to how your skin responds to the rice toner. If you notice any irritation, reduce the frequency of use or consider diluting it with water. Conversely, if your skin reacts positively, you can use it more frequently.

Consistency is Key:

To reap the full benefits of rice toner, consistency is key. Incorporate it into your routine regularly, and be patient – positive changes often occur over time with consistent use.

By incorporating these practical tips into your skincare routine, you can maximize the benefits of rice toner and achieve a healthier, more radiant complexion.

5.2 Guidance on When and How to Apply It for Optimal Results.

For optimal results, follow these guidelines on when and how to apply rice toner as part of your skincare routine:

When to Apply Rice Toner:

Morning Routine:

Use rice toner in the morning to refresh and prepare your skin for the day ahead.

It helps remove any impurities accumulated overnight and provides a clean canvas for makeup application.

Evening Routine:

Incorporate rice toner into your evening routine to aid in skin repair and rejuvenation. It helps remove the day's buildup and preps your skin for the application of serums or night creams.

After Cleansing:

Apply rice toner immediately after cleansing your face. Cleansing opens up your pores, allowing the toner to be absorbed more effectively.

Before Serum or Moisturizer:

Follow the toner with a serum or moisturizer to seal in the benefits. The toner enhances the absorption of subsequent products, maximizing their efficacy.

Throughout the Day (Optional):

If your skin tends to get dry or you need a quick pick-me-up, consider using a facial mist with rice toner throughout the day. This can help maintain hydration and freshness.

How to Apply Rice Toner:

Pour onto a Cotton Pad:

Pour a small amount of rice toner onto a cotton pad. Use enough to saturate the pad without dripping.

Swipe Gently Across Face:

Gently swipe the soaked cotton pad across your face in upward motions. Focus on areas where you want to address concerns, such as uneven skin tone or dry patches.

Pat onto Skin (Alternative):

Alternatively, pour a small amount of rice toner into clean hands and pat it onto your skin. This method is gentler and allows for even distribution without potential irritation from rubbing.

DIY Sheet Mask (Optional):

For a more intensive treatment, soak cotton pads or a compressed sheet mask with rice toner. Apply the mask to your face and leave it on for 10-15 minutes.

Avoid Eye Area:

Be cautious around the delicate eye area. Avoid applying toner directly to the eyes and instead focus on the cheeks, forehead, and chin.

Follow with Other Skincare Products:

After applying rice toner, follow up with your regular skincare routine. Apply serums, eye creams, and moisturizers to lock in the benefits.

Store Properly:

Store your rice toner in a cool, dark place, or refrigerate it for an added refreshing sensation during application.

Be Consistent:

Consistency is key for optimal results. Use rice toner regularly as part of your skincare routine to see long-term benefits.

By incorporating rice toner at the right times and using proper application techniques, you can enhance its effectiveness in promoting a healthier and more radiant complexion.

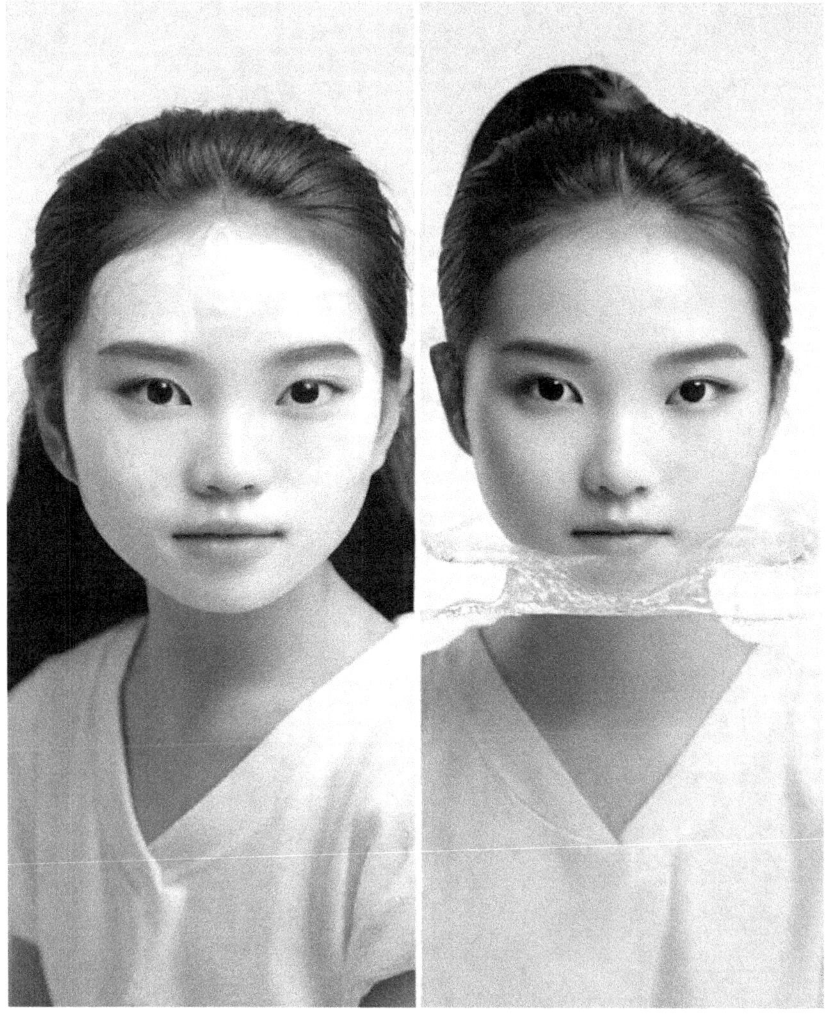

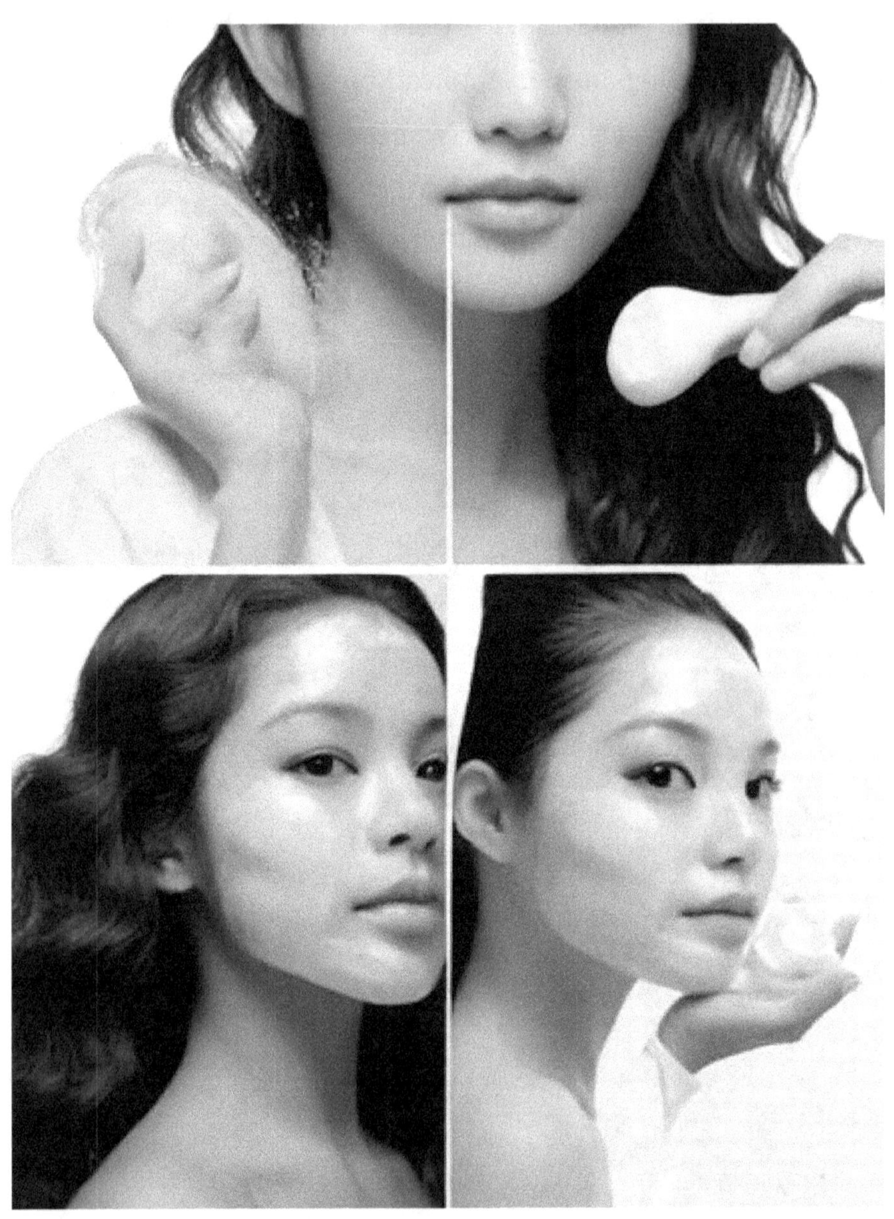

Chapter 6
Choosing the Right Rice Toner for Your Skin Type

6.1 Selecting the Most Suitable Rice Toner Based on Their Skin Type.

Selecting the most suitable rice toner for your skin type involves considering your specific skincare needs. Here's a guide to help readers choose the right rice toner based on their skin type:

1. For Dry Skin:

Recommended Ingredients: Look for rice toners with added moisturizing agents like glycerin or hyaluronic acid.

Additional Considerations: opt for formulations with nourishing oils like argan or jojoba for extra hydration.

2. For Oily or Acne-Prone Skin:

Recommended Ingredients: Choose rice toners with aloe vera for soothing properties and witch hazel for its astringent and acne-fighting benefits.

Additional Considerations: Tea tree oil, known for its antibacterial properties, can be beneficial for those prone to breakouts.

3. For Combination Skin:

Recommended Ingredients: Consider a balanced formula with both moisturizing and astringent properties.

Additional Considerations: Look for rice toners that contain green tea or chamomile for their calming effects on different areas of the face.

4. For Sensitive Skin:

Recommended Ingredients: opt for rice toners with soothing ingredients such as chamomile, calendula, or aloe vera.

Additional Considerations: Fragrance-free options and minimal ingredient lists can be gentler on sensitive skin.

5. For Aging or Mature Skin:

Recommended Ingredients: Choose rice toners with antioxidant-rich ingredients like green tea, along with those that contain peptides for anti-aging benefits.

Additional Considerations: Look for formulations with additional skincare powerhouse ingredients like rose water or collagen-boosting compounds.

6. For Dull or Uneven Skin Tone:

Recommended Ingredients: opt for rice toners that focus on brightening with ingredients like licorice extract or vitamin C.

Additional Considerations: Formulations with gentle exfoliants like rice enzymes can help improve skin texture and tone.

General Tips for All Skin Types:

Check the Ingredient List:

Review the ingredient list to ensure it aligns with your skin's needs. Avoid toners with potential irritants if you have sensitive skin.

Consider Additional Benefits:

Look for rice toners that offer additional benefits, such as anti-aging, hydration, or soothing properties, depending on your skincare goals.

Perform Patch Tests:

Before incorporating a new rice toner into your routine, perform a patch test to ensure your skin reacts positively.

Adjust Seasonally:

Consider adjusting your choice of rice toner based on seasonal changes. A more hydrating formula might be preferable in dry winter months, while a lighter option could be suitable for summer.

Be Patient:

Allow time for your skin to adjust and for the benefits of the rice toner to become noticeable. Consistency is key for optimal results.

By considering individual skin types and preferences, readers can make informed decisions when selecting a rice toner that aligns with their specific skincare needs and goals.

6.2 common concerns and considerations.

Addressing common concerns and considerations when using rice toner can help readers navigate potential challenges and optimize their skincare experience. Here are some key points to keep in mind:

1. Allergies and Sensitivities:

Concern: Some individuals may be allergic or sensitive to certain ingredients in rice toners.

Consideration: Always check the ingredient list and perform a patch test before widespread application. If irritation occurs, discontinue use and consult a dermatologist.

2. Acne and Breakouts:

Concern: Acne-prone individuals may worry about potential breakouts from using new products.

Consideration: Choose a rice toner with non-comedogenic ingredients. Look for formulations that include witch hazel or tea tree oil for acne-fighting properties.

3. Over-Exfoliation:

Concern: Excessive exfoliation, even with gentle rice toners, can lead to irritation.

Consideration: Use rice toner as directed and avoid combining it with other exfoliating products to prevent over-exfoliation.

If using a toner with exfoliating properties, limit use to a few times per week.

4. Hydration Levels:

Concern: Dry or dehydrated skin may need additional hydration beyond what a rice toner provides.

Consideration: Follow the rice toner with a suitable moisturizer to lock in hydration. Consider using a more emollient formulation during drier seasons.

5. Choosing the Right Type:

Concern: Readers may feel overwhelmed by the variety of rice toners available on the market.

Consideration: Select a rice toner based on your specific skin type and concerns. Consider additional ingredients in the toner that address particular skincare goals.

6. Patch Testing:

Concern: Neglecting to patch test can lead to unexpected reactions.

Consideration: Perform a patch test on a small area of skin before using the rice toner on your face. This helps identify any potential adverse reactions.

7. Storage and Shelf Life:

Concern: Improper storage may impact the efficacy of the toner.

Consideration: Store the rice toner in a cool, dark place, or refrigerate it for an added refreshing sensation. Be mindful of the product's shelf life and discard if it expires.

8. Consistency in Usage:

Concern: Inconsistent use may hinder desired results.

Consideration: Incorporate the rice toner consistently into your routine for best results. Find a frequency that works for you, whether it's daily or a few times a week.

9. Potential for Irritation:

Concern: Some individuals may experience irritation, particularly if they have sensitive skin.

Consideration: Choose a rice toner with minimal ingredients and avoid products with potential irritants. If irritation persists, discontinue use and consult with a skincare professional.

10. Adapting to Seasonal Changes:

Concern: Skin needs may vary with seasonal changes.

Consideration: Adjust your choice of rice toner based on seasonal conditions. A more hydrating formula may be suitable for dry winters, while a lighter option may be preferred in humid summers.

Addressing these common concerns and considerations empowers you to use rice toner effectively and integrate it seamlessly into their skincare routines while minimizing potential challenges.

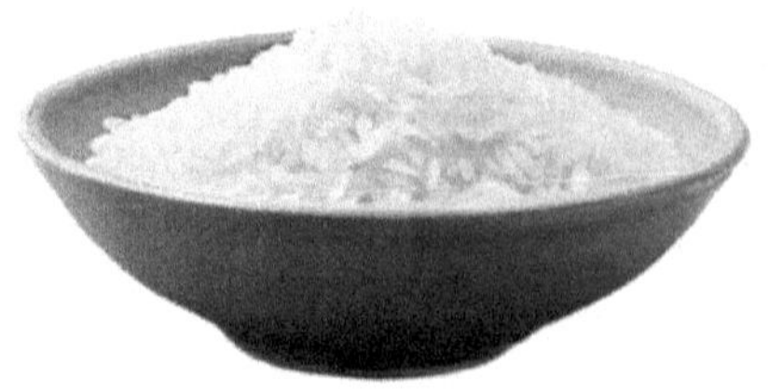

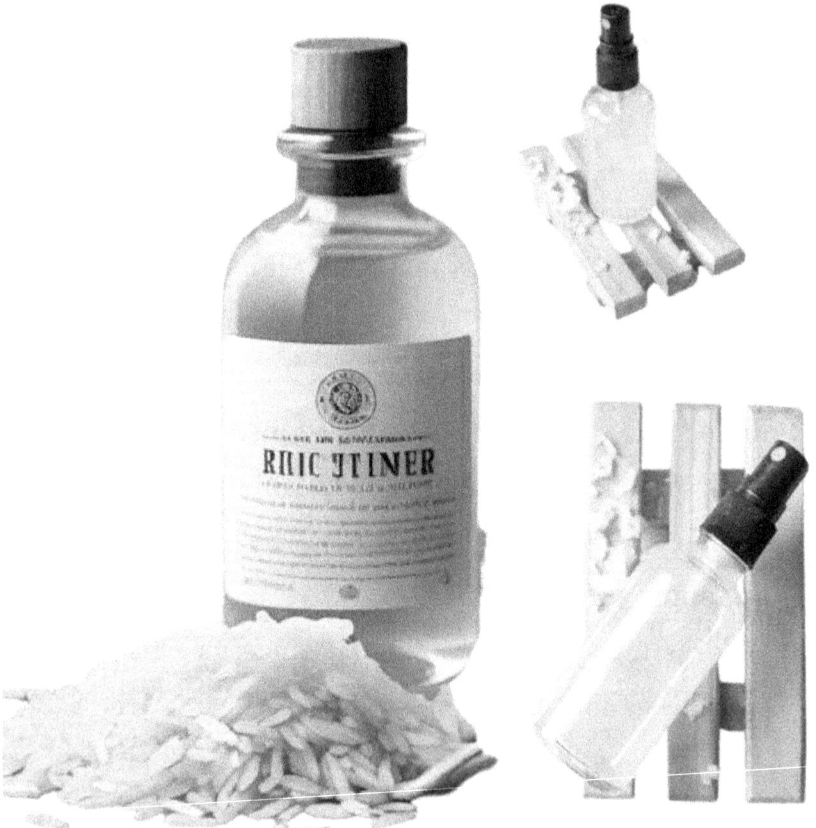

Chapter 7
Quick Facts Recap

7.1 The Key Quick Facts Presented in This Book.

In "Rice Toner 101: Quick Facts for Glowing Skin," readers will discover a wealth of information highlighting the benefits and versatility of incorporating rice toner into their skincare routines. Here's a summarized overview of the key quick facts presented in the book:

Historical Roots: Explore the ancient beauty practices that inspired the use of rice toner, particularly in Asian cultures, showcasing its enduring legacy in skincare traditions.

Scientific Efficacy: Understand the science behind the effectiveness of rice toner, delving into its nutrient-rich composition, antioxidant properties, and capacity for moisture retention.

Diverse Benefits: Uncover the multifaceted benefits of rice toner, including its ability to brighten the complexion, provide deep hydration, soothe sensitive skin, and contribute to an even skin tone.

Types of Rice Toners: Navigate the diverse landscape of rice toner products, from traditional rice water toners to fermented variations, catering to a range of skincare needs and preferences.

DIY Delights: Unlock the secrets of creating rice toner at home with simple and effective DIY recipes, allowing readers to customize formulations based on their skin types.

Application Mastery: Learn practical tips and techniques for seamlessly integrating rice toner into daily skincare routines, optimizing its benefits for radiant and healthy skin.

Choosing the Perfect Fit: Gain insights into selecting the right rice toner based on individual skin types, addressing common concerns, and maximizing results.

Recap and Reinforce: Summarize the key quick facts, reinforcing the compelling reasons to make rice toner a staple in skincare regimens, emphasizing its natural and gentle approach to achieving glowing and healthy skin.

Through these quick facts, the book aims to empower readers with comprehensive knowledge, enabling them to make informed decisions about incorporating rice toner into their skincare rituals for a radiant and revitalized complexion.

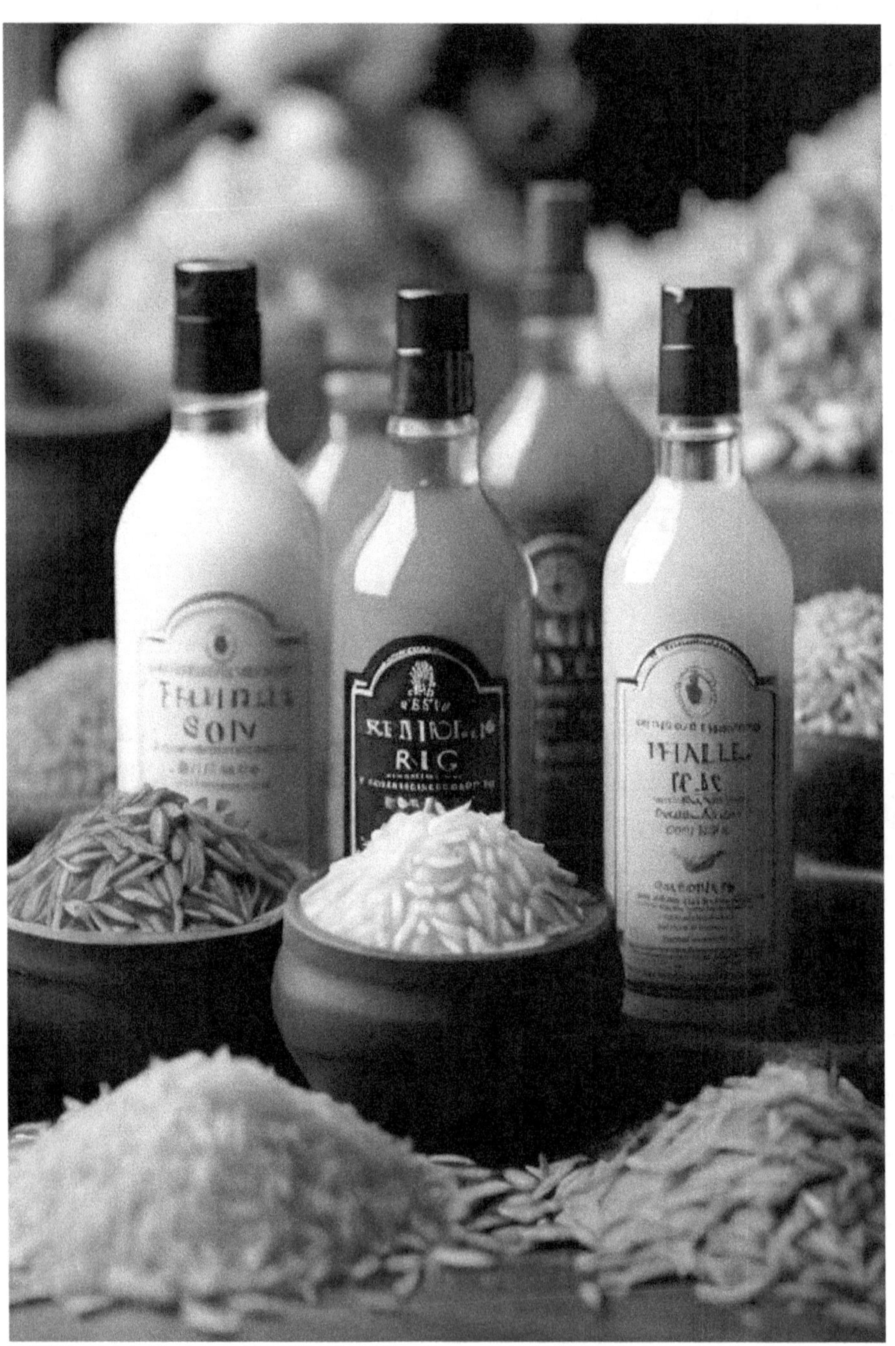

Conclusion

The Importance of Incorporating Rice Toner into A Skincare Routine.

Using rice toner in your skincare routine offers a multitude of benefits that contribute to achieving glowing and healthy skin. Reinforcing these benefits emphasizes the compelling reasons to make rice toner a staple in your daily regimen:

Radiant Complexion:

Reinforcement: Rice toner's brightening properties contribute to a luminous complexion, diminishing dullness and leaving your skin with a healthy, radiant glow.

Hydration Boost:

Reinforcement: The natural moisturizing elements in rice toner provide a hydration boost, preventing dryness and maintaining supple, nourished skin.

Antioxidant Defense:

Reinforcement: Packed with antioxidants, rice toner acts as a formidable defense against free radicals, preserving the skin's youthful appearance and protecting against premature aging.

Soothing and Calming:

Reinforcement: Ideal for sensitive skin, rice toner's soothing properties alleviate irritation and redness, providing a gentle and calming effect.

Even Skin Tone:

Reinforcement: The potential exfoliating enzymes in rice toner contribute to a smoother and more even skin tone, addressing hyperpigmentation and uneven texture.

Versatility for All Skin Types:

Reinforcement: Regardless of your skin type—oily, dry, combination, or sensitive—rice toner's versatility makes it suitable for everyone, offering a universal solution for a diverse range of skincare needs.

Prepares Skin for Further Products:

Reinforcement: By using rice toner before applying serums, moisturizers, or other treatments, you optimize your skincare routine, ensuring better absorption and enhanced efficacy of subsequent products.

Natural and Gentle:

Reinforcement: One of the standout features of rice toner is its natural and gentle nature, providing an effective yet mild option for those seeking a botanical approach to skincare.

By reinforcing these benefits, users are encouraged to recognize the transformative potential of rice toner in achieving and maintaining glowing, healthy skin. Integrating this simple yet powerful step into your skincare routine contributes to a radiant complexion and an overall sense of skin well-being.

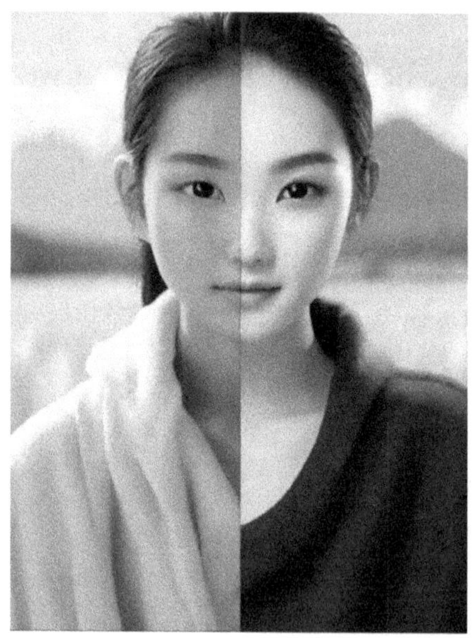

Dear Readers,

Embarking on a journey to discover the beauty and wellness benefits of rice toner can be a transformative and rewarding experience for your skin. As you delve into the world of skincare enriched by the natural essence of rice, we encourage you to explore and enjoy the multitude of benefits that await you:

Radiant Glow Awaits:

Experience the joy of unveiling a radiant complexion as the brightening properties of rice toner work their magic, leaving your skin with a luminous and healthy glow.

Indulge in Deep Hydration:

Immerse yourself in the deep hydration offered by rice toner, reveling in the sensation of supple and nourished skin. Let each application be a moment of self-care and hydration.

Defend Your Beauty:

Embrace the antioxidant-rich shield of rice toner, safeguarding your skin against environmental stressors. Witness the preservation of your skin's youthful vitality and the defense against premature aging.

Soothe and Calm:

Allow the soothing properties of rice toner to caress your skin, alleviating irritation and redness. Let this gentle embrace be a source of comfort and tranquility for your sensitive skin.

Revel in Even Skin Tone:

Delight in the journey towards a smoother and more even skin tone. Let the exfoliating enzymes of rice toner unveil a canvas that reflects your natural beauty.

Versatility for Every Skin Type:

Regardless of your skin type, let the versatility of rice toner be your skincare ally. Explore its adaptability, finding the perfect match for your unique skin needs.

Prepare for Beauty Unveiled:

Prepare your skin for a showcase of beauty by incorporating rice toner into your routine. Witness the enhanced absorption and efficacy of subsequent skincare products, making each step a celebration of your skin's well-being.

Embrace Nature's Gentleness:

Revel in the natural and gentle touch of rice toner, a botanical symphony that harmonizes with your skin. Let this simplicity be a source of joy in your skincare ritual.

Embark on this journey with curiosity and enthusiasm, discovering the wonders that rice toner can unfold for your skin.

May each application be a celebration of self-love, allowing you to indulge in the beauty and benefits that await you.

Here's to radiant and healthy skin, and the joy of embracing your natural glow!

With warm regards,

[A J BLAZING]

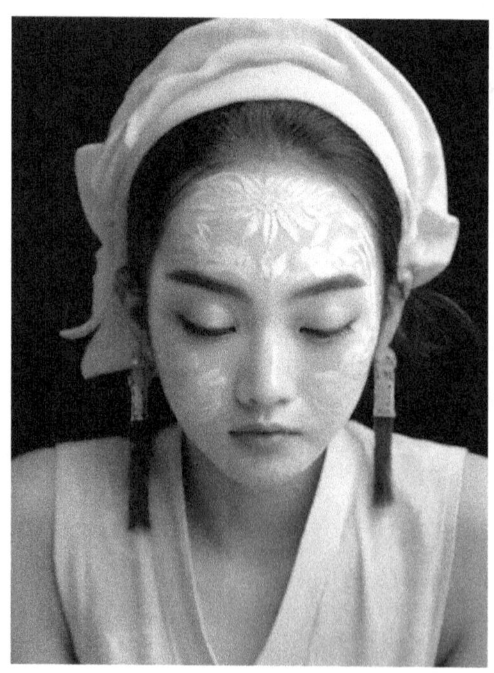